FUCK IT, I'M FAT

FUCK IT, I'M FAT
MY WEIGHT LOSS JOURNEY

BY

JULIA PRESS-SIMMONS

www.myspace.com/ragewriter

www.facebook.com/julia.p.simmons

www.twitter.com/jpsimmons

Published by Queen Midas Books
Copyright © 2012 by Julia Press Simmons
Cover design by: Genesis Graphix

First Printing July 2012
Printed in the United States of America
10 9 8 7 6 5 4 3 2 1

DISCLAIMER

These ideas and suggestions written by Julia Press Simmons are provided as general educational information only and should not be construed as medical advice or care. All matters regarding your health require supervision by a personal physician or other appropriate health professional familiar with your current health status. Always consult your personal physican before making any dietary or exercise changes. Julia Press Simmons, and Royalty Press disclaim any liability or warranties of any kind arising directly or indirectly from use of this information. If any medical problems develop, always consult your personal physician. Only your physician can provide you medical advice.

Throughout this document are links to external sites. These external sites contain information created and maintained by other individuals and organizations and are provided for the user's convenience. Julia Press Simmons, and Royalty Press do not control nor can they guarantee the accuracy, relevance, timeliness, or completeness of this information. Neither is it intended to endorse any view expressed nor reflect its importance by inclusion in this book.

ACKNOWLEDGEMENTS

I knew this book would come out this year, because of all the love in my life. My mother's guidance, counsel, and permission gave me the strength to face my truth. My son's partnership truly lightened my load, and his father's friendship strengthened my resolve.

I have to extend a special thanks to my editor. Nora, I am truly blessed to have you work on this project with me. Thank you for the patience and extreme care you exhibited. I owe the polish and professionalism to you. You is one bad ass mofo from the windy city!

To Junnita Jackson my brand manager extraordinaire, thank you for late night calls and early morning vids. Thanks always putting our friendship before our business. Thanks for being my big sister and best friend.

TABLE OF CONTENTS

DEDICATIONS

THIS BOOK IS FOR MY READERS

THANK YOU AND I LOVE YOU ALL!

INTRODUCTION

Dear Readers,

I must have started this book hundreds of times over the last few years, but could never bring myself to complete it until now. I'm no longer afraid to face the truth. I'm 34 years old and I have a wicked food addiction and a serious lack of impulse control. They say the first step on the road to recovery is admitting you have a problem. Whoop, here it is. Thank you all so much for the love and support.

Yours truly,

Julia

Mission…

MY BIG AND SEXY HAS BECOME BIG AND DEADLY

Well, actually, it has been deadly for quite some time. I was diagnosed with diabetes in 2005, but I've been fat-as-fuck since forever. I've lived a hard life, and food has always been my source of comfort. Whenever I'd go through something, anything, I'd eat, and eat, and eat. It didn't matter if I was full, I didn't eat to get full, I ate to feel better and it never ever worked.

Layout…

I am going to attempt to outline the major turning points of my addiction and couple it with what I've learned about my disease and proper eating habits over the years. Each chapter contains a snapshot of my life and a lesson on positive food choices, healthy eating habits, and life style changes. This book is not an admission of defeat, it's a testimony. I constantly struggle with my weight and illness mostly in silence or with dry wit, however I can't any longer. I'm writing this book for therapeutic purposes. I wanted to spell it out for myself and others who struggle with obesity. This is me trying to get it right!

I CHANGED A FEW NAMES AND PLACES TO PROTECT THE PEOPLE WHO MAY NOT WANT THEIR PART IN MY STORY TOLD.

Chapter 1 – The Beginning

The loneliest part of my childhood was on Clifford Street. We moved there two years after my sister Denise passed away. Two of my brothers were in prison and my oldest brother was living in New Jersey doing his own thing. My father owned a bar on Montgomery Avenue, and my mother worked second shift as a housekeeper downtown.

It seemed like I was always by myself. My parents were sleeping when I left for school in the morning and were at work when I got home. I learned early on that friends who make fun of you and make you feel bad all the time aren't really friends. I became depressed with that little piece of wisdom and started keeping to myself.

That didn't help the lonely situation at all.

I was thirteen years old and miserable beyond belief. This is when I started to put on weight. I would come home from school, plop a tape in the VCR and make myself a meal. I'd do this three, or four times a night. I didn't know what I was doing. I wasn't mature enough to know that I was using the food to feel better, although I remember the moment I figured it all out.

I walked home from school with a crowd of girls that hated my guts trailing behind me.

"You're a dirty bitch," one of the girls in the crowd hollered.

Everything in me screamed to run, but I forced myself to walk steady. I was supposed to fight Linda. That's why the angry mob was following me. Everyone wanted front row seats for my ass whooping.

Earlier that day I was walking up to the teacher's desk to turn in my report and Linda pointed out that I had had the same jeans on for three days. The class erupted in laughter and my heart nosedived into my stomach.

Without hesitation I stopped dead in my tracks, turned towards Linda, and threw my hands on my hips. "I can change these jeans, but you can't change a damn thing about your crackhead momma or cracked-up face."

"Your face does look like ass crack, Linda," hollered a boy from the back of the class.

The laughter and the humiliation instantly shifted from me to her. I high fived a few people before dropping my report on Mr. Lee's desk, and switching back to my seat. I looked at Linda with a self-satisfied smirk, and the look she shot back at me gave me chills.

She mouthed the words, "I'm gonna fuck you up."

The glint in her eyes made my blood run cold. Way to go, Julie, I thought with a shudder. Way to go. It was now a quarter to three and I was desperately trying to make it home before she beat the living shit out of me. I looked at the twisted tree that sat on the corner of my block and smiled. I was almost there— almost home.

I turned the corner and pain exploded in my shoulder. I stumbled, fell, and the crowd formed a tight ring around me. Linda kicked, punched and slapped me until I was black and blue. I laid there until they left. Not one person helped me up. I was on the corner of my block and it took me forty-five minutes to get home.

This memory is seared in my brain. I can close my eyes and see it as if it happened yesterday.

Something profound changed in me that day. I became a little cynical. I tasted depression for the first time. I cried until my head hurt. I took those jeans off and threw them in the trash. I went into the kitchen and pulled out the turkey my mother made for Sunday dinner. I cut off a big hunk and ate it right there. I sobbed and choked and ate until my tears dried up. I started to feel better with each bite. My stomach was starting to hurt a little bit, but I kept on eating.

Things started to look up a few months after that. My mom's friend had a break-in at her house and she came to stay with us for a bit.

Then, BAM, I wasn't lonely anymore. All of a sudden I had a big sister who was home when my parents were not. She had an awesome record collection. She would put on classic R&B while she cleaned up the house and made dinner. She treated me like a Barbie doll, always dressing me up and fixing my hair. Loneliness was a thing of the past especially when my father's bar closed down.

He bought the business home, literally. I felt as though I lived in the middle of a late night movie. I had a new big sister and tons of people around. They played cards in the kitchen, danced to old records in the dining room and rolled joints and told stories in the living room. Life just couldn't get any better, as far as I was concerned.

I was truly happy for a few months. Then one day school let out early, I don't really remember why, I just remember that was the day the happiness left my house. I came home and found my new big sister, my mom's best friend, in bed with my father. I wanted to tell my mother, but I didn't know how. I was conflicted; I loved all three of them. Withdrawing from life, I ate more, and slept more. The late-night movie and the fairytale life came to an abrupt end.

They flaunted their affair in front of everyone except my mother. The neighborhood kids started to tease me. Life was back to its regular hell. A few months into the inferno, my little brother was born - not to my mother, but to her friend.

The cat was out of the bag, and my mother made my father choose. For the time being, he chose us and we moved to New Jersey.

I ate all of that pain.

CRBOCRBOCRBOCRBOCRBOCRBOCRBOCRBO

- How Not To Be Fat

Because I know how to be fat, I got that shit down to a science.

By the time I turned 25, I was really good at hiding my eating problem. I ate like a bird in public and would blame my continuous weight gain on a slow metabolism. Funny thing about that excuse was I really had no fucking clue about my metabolism at all. I couldn't tell you if it was slow, fast or middling. I must have heard and used the word metabolism a million times before I knew what it meant. I think I heard Oprah say it on her show way back when and ran with it.

Webster's Definition:

Metabolism - the sum of the processes in the buildup and destruction of protoplasm; specifically: the chemical changes in living cells by which energy is provided for vital processes and activities and new material is assimilated...

Translation:

Metabolism - Energy level. It keeps you going. It burns off calories. It works all day and all night, although it does slow down when you're sleeping. Your metabolism is the body's engine. It keeps shit in motion.

*As you age, your body tends to lose muscle and gain fat which slows down your ability to burn calories. This is one of the driving forces behind my decision to get serious about my weight loss. It is much easier to lose weight when you are younger than when you get older, point blank period. And, baby, I ain't getting' no younger! Your metabolism relies on fuel to keep it going. And the earlier in the day you get your metabolism going, the more calories you burn off during the course of the day. This is why we are often told that breakfast is the most important meal of the day.

That's where I fuck up on the regular. I mean I eat breakfast (I don't skip any meals), but I usually eat something light at breakfast and throughout the day and then pig-the-hell-out at night. I've learned that boosting your metabolism isn't enough to lose weight. You also have to decrease you caloric intake. This reduction should be discussed with a doctor and/or a nutritionist, because every single food on the planet has a different make-up. Calorie consumption is not a one-size-fits-all situation, but I'll talk about that more in the next chapter.

*The source for everything marked with an asterisk can be found at the end of the book.

Chapter 2 – PUPPY LOVE

Puberty and the extra pounds helped to produce one brick shithouse of a body on a 15-year-old. I could not walk down the street without turning a head or eliciting a cat call. The onslaught of new attention was a happy distraction from the soap opera home life.

Before we left for Jersey, I met a really handsome older boy. I'll call him Harry (not his real name). It was my birthday and my mother agreed to let me have a slumber party. I had a couple of girlfriends from the science club come over. My mom and dad had to work second shift, so they left us money to get a pizza. We got dressed up like we were going to the hottest night club just to pick it up.

Walking over the bridge was an adventure back in the day, because North Philly was a tangle of feuding neighborhoods. Not necessarily a rival to the gang wars of old, but it was definitely cliquish and territorial. We were very excited and looking for a little trouble.

It didn't take a long time for us to find it.

Harry and his brothers stopped us on the way back from the pizza joint. Score! When Harry walked over to me, I thought this was by far the best birthday bash I'd ever had. He was handsome and tall with a sleek, muscular build. He pulled me to the side and actually stuttered while asking my name and number. He had a deep, dark chocolate complexion with a dazzling white smile that boasted cute dimples. I was charmed down to my toes. My girlfriends literally had to pull me away. We raced home just to get on the phone and call the boys we had just met.

This was the beginning of my personal nightmare. I often think back and wonder how so much pain could be born of such sweet innocence.

We had ourselves a whirlwind romance that was magnified by super-strong adolescent emotions. I needed to see him every day and talk to him every night. Before I knew what was happening, young Harry had become my life. The night before we moved to New Jersey I broke my curfew for the very first time. I spent the night on the Montgomery Avenue Bridge professing my undying love. This happened over twenty years ago, but it is crystal clear in my memory.

He held me so close that I could feel his heartbeat against my breast.

"I love you, Moe," he said softly in my ear.

My heart broke into a thousand tiny pieces. My parents were going to move me from the only person in the world that mattered. "I love you, too, Harry."

He kissed me slowly at first, teasing his lips against mine. My body tingled against his and a soft moan escaped my lips. His kiss turned feral at that moment, and I was introduced to true desire and passion. His hands were everywhere—under my shirt, down my pants. My body was his playground, and I liked it.

I wanted to give myself to him right there on the bridge. All he had to do was ask and I would have stripped in public. Hours passed before we finally pulled apart. He walked me to the corner of my block and kissed me softly on the cheek before saying good-bye. He had tears in his eyes and my heart in his hands.

I remember walking away from him was the hardest thing imaginable, but I managed. I was three hours pass my curfew and I gave less than a fuck about it. We were leaving in the morning, and in my mind there was nothing that my parents could do to me that was worse than moving me to another state.

By the time I slid my key into the front door tears were running down my face like river rapids. I swung the door open slowly and almost had a heart attack when I saw my mother sitting in the living room. Her face was contorted in a look of pure pain that mirrored how I felt. I opened my mouth to deliver my alibi but she held her hand up to silence me.

"Are you still a virgin?" she asked quietly.

I was shocked by the question, but I answered it instantly. "Yes, I am a virgin."

She stared at me for a full minute trying to gauge whether or not I was being truthful. Finally she sighed, stood up, and stretched. "You better go upstairs and get some rest. We've got a big day tomorrow."

***

Leaving Harry was hard. Living in a new city with silent parents was harder. My father gave me more money to compensate for the lack of love and happiness in our home. I was cool with that. I used the extra money to fuel my budding habit.

There was a small grocery store two blocks from our new house, and I became their biggest junk food customer. I'd hit them hard in the morning before school, and I'd hit them low after.

Food was my only friend.

My father let me make long distant calls to Philly on Fridays, and I called Harry. I'd become obsessed with the thought of him meeting another girl and me losing the only person who gave a shit about me. He promised that he wouldn't, but I was still terrified. I broke up with him as some sort of weirdo self-protection mechanism. He was going to leave me, so I'd leave him first.

Perfect 15-year-old logic…

Heartbroken, young Harry decides to walk over to New Jersey from North Philly, and I rewarded him with my virginity. The entire dynamic of our relationship changed. Who knew that sex would be the worst possible thing for an emotionally unstable young girl with a habit of overeating?

I'm not going to recount my first sexual experience but I will tell you the effects.

I cried all the time. My insecurities multiplied and Harry became more important to me than air. The more I yearned for him, the more he pulled away. My grades began to drop, and my eating increased. I gained twenty pounds. I withdrew into my shell. I stopped talking. I stopped dreaming, and for a time, I stopped writing.

After a few short months my father convinced my mother to move us back to Philly. I didn't know how he managed to do that, but I was happy as hell about it. The distance between Harry and I was killing me and moving back to Philly was all I wanted out of life at that time.

Not!

ⒸⓈⒸⓈⒸⓈⒸⓈⒸⓈⒸⓈⒸⓈⒸⓈ

-Eating to Live

Because I got living to eat down pat!

I attended nursing clinicals at Harrisburg Area Community College. Nutrition was one of the modules of Nursing 101. I remember sitting in class at one of Professor Lieb's lectures. The topic of discussion was caloric intake. A calorie is a unit of energy. Go to the Website How Stuff Works for the complete scientific breakdown of how calories work, because I'm just going to tell you what I learned about them in relation to getting the spare truck tire from around my middle.

The amount of calories that you need to take in each day depends upon your height, your gender, your body type and your activity level. There are hundreds of different calorie consumption guides online that will teach you how many calories you should be consuming each day based upon these factors. I like to use the "Calorie Calculator" at freedieting.com, because you don't have to sign up for anything on the site and they do all the math for you. There are usually three choices when it comes to activity level - sedentary (which means that you do not exercise much at all), semi-active and very active.

A rough example:

When you find the amount of calories that you need for your body, cut it by 200 calories. If the calculator tells me that I need to consume 1800 calories a day based upon my height, sex, body type and activity level, I'll cut it to 1600 calories a day. My instructor explained that I could speed up my weight loss process without making a dramatic change in the amount of food I eat. Armed with Google, I can now find out how many calories are in whatever I choose to put in my mouth. I am also thankful for the calorie info on every fast food menu I see.

Here are my numbers:

Age: 35
Weight: 282lbs (It hurts me to type that)
Height: 5'2"
Exercise Level: 3 times per week
The Calorie Calculator tells me that to maintain this weight I need to consume 2654 calories per day and to lose weight safely (1 to 2 pounds per week) I need to consume 2256 calories per day

Chapter 3 - Striking Distance

I thought about starting this chapter off by telling you about the first time Harry hit me, but I decided that story was irrelevant. We were young and immature in an adult relationship; he hit me and I hit him right back. The real story, the one that I believe speaks more to the purpose of this book, is the day I stopped fighting back.

I was in the tenth grade when it happened. The weight gain from overeating continued to fill out my adolescent body. I could barely fit any of the clothes in my closet, and what I could fit made me look like I was fittin' to walk the ho stroll. I remember coming home from school wearing a pair of stone washed jeans that were practically bursting at the seams. This year, stopping traffic and turning heads was the norm. After I became sexually active, the more attention I received, the harder I strutted.

"Damn, girl, your ass is about to break out of those jeans. Come here and let me holler at you for a minute."

I smiled over my shoulder at him. "No," I said with a giggle. The man looked old enough to be my father.

He jogged over to me and grabbed my arm. I laughed and jerked away from him.

"Girl, for real, I could fall in love with you. What's your name?"

"My name is Ms. I-Got-a-Man."

He laughed. "Alright, Ms. Got-a-Man; I won't tell him if you won't."

Smiling, I shook my head and walked away. I loved the attention and commotion my curves caused. However, I had no idea that Harry was watching the whole exchange from across the street. I forgot that he told me he was going to walk me home. I was almost there when he hit me.

He slapped the shit out of me and the force of the blow spun me around. Pain exploded in the side of my face. I couldn't think or react. I had never been hit so hard in my life. There was a look of complete rage on his face. His eyes blazed and his eyebrows knitted together to form an angry line. The corner of his mouth was curled up in a snarl.

I stumbled into the street and barely caught my balance before hitting the hot tar. "Nigga, what's wrong with you?"

He didn't respond. Instead, he followed me into the street and punched me in the face. My head snapped back so hard that a spasm shot straight down my spine. My face felt like it was going to explode. He walked over to me and I threw my hands up to guard against another blow. But, he didn't hit me; he helped me to my feet.

He laughed. "Girl, you are clumsy as hell." He brushed my jeans off as bright red blood dripped from my nose onto my t-shirt.

I was confused until I saw the people walking pass. The woman headed towards me, but the man she was with pulled her away. "That's not your business," he said loudly. I locked eyes with her and silently pleaded for help, but she put her head down and walked away.

My heart sank to my knees. Normally, I would fight him back. I would swing wildly and curse him out. Not this time. I was too afraid. The pain was blinding. I didn't want to fight. I wanted to go home.

Harry tugged me onto the pavement. "If you want to be a skank, and wear skanky shit, I'm gonna treat you like one."

This is the moment that I was introduced to fear. I've been afraid before, many, many times before, but not to this degree. I followed him because I didn't want to hurt anymore. I didn't know that the pain I was heading towards was much worse than the pain that had been dished out.

He took me deep into the park. It seemed as if we walked for hours, but I know that it was just twenty minutes or so. My tears and blood had dried up on my face, but my spirit was still weeping. I remember feeling hopeless. I wasn't used to that.

He stopped in a clearing not far from the river and Kelly Drive. I could hear the traffic but I couldn't see through the trees. He took off his shirt and turned to face me.

"Who else are you fucking?"

I looked at him in pure shock. I opened my mouth to say no one, but he punched me in my stomach before I could get the words out. I fell to my knees gasping for air. Tears stung in my eyes. I want to go home, I thought. He pulled my hair and yanked my head back.

"If you want to be a skank, I'm going to treat you like one." He pushed me down on the ground and kicked me in my side. "Turn around," he said between clenched teeth, but I couldn't move. He stooped down and flipped me over.

"Stop," I cried. I could barely see through my tears. He moved and I brought my hands up instinctively to shield myself. He didn't hit me again. He did something much, much worse, and the memory of it, the savagery took years to overcome.

When he undid my pants, I wanted to fight, but the pain in my face and side was excruciating. If I had had any idea how damaging the pain of being raped by someone you loved was, I would have fought with all my heart and soul. It didn't last long. He ripped inside of me with the same speed and brutality he had showed moments before. I looked at the trees and the grass because I couldn't bear to look at him. When he was finished he collapsed on top of me and began to cry. The last of my innocence was gone.

I had to sit in the bathtub for hours, heating up the water every so often. I cried until I had no more tears. I washed five times and still felt dirty. The next day, no one noticed the bruises and cuts on my face and arms. I ditched school for weeks and ate everything I could get my hands on. I felt dead inside and nothing I did took the pain away. I was ashamed, confused and lonely, so lonely.

Some days I would sit across from my father while he watched TV and pray for him to ask me what was wrong because I had promised myself to tell if someone asked. If anyone suspected, I would tell them everything. My eating became out of control. I would binge and get sick. My stomach hurt all the time. I wanted to tell someone about it, but I was more ashamed of that than being raped.

I think I didn't tell anyone because I felt I would be telling on myself. Is it really rape when it's your boyfriend? I didn't say no or fight back. What if I got in trouble? I decided that being silent and forgetting about it was the best thing I could do.

My parents were either working hard or too wrapped up in their own drama to notice my pain. I had no friends and the bulk of my family lived in Jersey. When Harry showed up at my school to talk, I was happy. Somebody cared. I missed him.

"I'm sorry," he said with tears in his eyes. "I'll never hit you again. I'll never hurt you again." A single tear fell from his eyes. "I understand if you don't want to see me again. I can't even bear to look at myself."

I wiped the tear from his face.

"I understand if you don't want to be with me. I love you so much." His tears fell rapidly then and he had a look of fear in his eye.

"I don't think us being together is a good idea," I said softly. I remember wanting to hold him. The urge was overwhelming.

"Okay," he said standing to his full height. "I understand. I'm not good enough for you anyway. If you won't be with me, I really don't have anything left to live for." He turned to walk away and my heart thudded against my chest.

"Wait, what do you mean?" I raced to catch up with him. He told me how no one loved him or gave a shit about what happened to him. His words echoed in my head and my heart. We felt the same way.

"I care about you," I said softly. He grabbed me and held me very tight. We went back to my house and made love on the living room floor while my parents were at work.

I needed to be loved so badly that I took it from the one person who hurt me the most.

We were back together and, in my naivety, I believed that we were stronger, closer for having been through that horror. Days turned into weeks, and weeks morphed into months, and Harry and I were inseparable. I got pregnant in October of 1992.

I was 15 years old. They didn't make enough hoagies in Philadelphia to get me through this.

CRBOCRBOCRBOCRBOCRBOCRBOCRBO

Fast foods:

I have a love-hate relationship with McDonald's. Before I started writing full time, I worked twelve to sixteen hours a day. I got used to eating at fast food restaurants several times a shift. One of the nurses that I worked with told me that I was slowly killing myself. She said that one meal from McDonald's was about the total amount of calories that I should have for the entire day. I decided to look into the nutritional facts for myself and went to the McDonald's Website to find out more. My favorite lunch included the Big Mac, which contains 550 calories, a medium order of fries, which has 380 calories, and a medium Coke with 210 calories. That is over 1100 calories and I would eat like that several times a day. It is much easier to control your calorie consumption if you prepare your food at home.

If you do eat out, grab a salad that is packed with plenty of leafy greens and baked or grilled chicken. Use a low-fat or fat free dressing, but remember that pre-packaged dressings can be loaded with sugar. A friend of mind suggests that you use all dressings sparingly - instead of drenching a fast food salad in the whole packet of dressing, dip forkfuls of salad in a cup of dressing on the side to gauge the amount you're consuming. I try to remember that I'm watching my calories and try not to go over my limit. Fast food puts me at close to my calorie limit mighty, um, well, fast.

Fried Foods

I know fried food is the bomb-dot-com, but it just isn't good for you and is loaded with fat and calories. I had to ask myself, Is eating fried chicken worth being sick and tired all the time, Julia? The answer is no, plain and simple. * When food is fried its nutritional content changes—the food loses water and takes up fat, increasing its energy density or calories. Refrying or reusing oil causes food to lose unsaturated fat and gain trans-fat. *Trans-fat increases bad cholesterol which can lead to heart disease

In a perfect world, I'd swear off all fried foods forever, but sometimes I get a hankering for it. If you must fry try sunflower oil. Kyrsty Hazell of the Huffington Post highlighted a study that shows how oils extracted from plants are less harmful to the cardiovascular system.

Processed Foods, Frozen Meals and Condiments

Every single person who tried to stage an intervention for my junk food addiction has warned me about the dangers of eating processed foods. But how the hell do you do that when almost all food is processed these days? I have found that the answer lies in the ingredients. There are levels to food processing and you can figure out the level by checking the label. The closer the food is to its organic state, the better. If the ingredients contain a bunch of chemicals that I can't pronounce, I don't put it in my mouth.

Travis Stork, MD, host of The Doctors on television and author of the book "The Lean Belly Prescription," says processed foods are also high in calories, filled with hidden sugar, excessive salt, and other health saboteurs that can ruin your diet. "Sodium shows up in canned soups, salad dressings, and even products that don't immediately come to mind when we think of 'salty' foods, such as pasta, bread and cereals," said Rachel Johnson, Ph.D., R.D., a professor of nutrition at the University of Vermont and a volunteer for the American Heart Association. I've decided that making my own food won't kill me, and it might just help me live a little longer.

Ordinary table condiments like ketchup, mayonnaise and mustard can also be loaded with sugar, fat or salt. Of course, a little won't kill any diet, and a little mayonnaise isn't the devil, either, as fat can be satisfying. I would recommend using condiments sparingly, of course.

On the flip side, all processed foods aren't bad. Web MD has a comparative list of healthy frozen dinners, and Shereen Jegtvig wrote an article at about.com on the *benefits of some processed foods. She claims that freezing fruits and vegetables preserves their vitamins and minerals and makes them convenient to store, cook and eat all year around.

Sweets

Now on to my weakness ... I love all cakes, cookies, pastries, donuts, and any kind of candy, but they are all bursting with empty calories. They offer no nutritional value and will leave you feeling hungry. They are a total waste of time, can wreck your diet, and make you feel bad. Nancy Appleton, author of "Lick the Sugar Habit," claims that too much sugar in your diet can cause food allergies, endocrine problems, hypoglycemia, diabetes, tooth decay, osteoporosis, arthritis, cancer, and many other degenerative diseases. If you need to have something sweet to top off your meal, as some people do, then have something like a mint or a small piece of hard candy. A square of dark chocolate will do, as well. Be sure to count this in with your calorie intake.

Chapter 4 – Postpartum Depression

I told my father that I was pregnant before I told my mother. It was easier that way. My mother was the disciplinarian. She held very high standards for me, and I feared disappointing her more than I feared death. My father was more like a friend. He never seemed to get mad at me for anything and he approved of my relationship with Harry. That fact didn't stop me from being nervous about telling him, but it made it a little easier.

So, bright and early one Saturday morning, I sat my father down at the kitchen table over two bowls of Frosted Flakes and bananas. "Daddy," I said, pushing the cereal around with my spoon, "I'm pregnant."

My father pushed his bowl away and stared at me. I put my head down in shame.

He cleared his throat and sat back in his chair. "Julie, you know sex is about the best thing in the world besides ice cream."

I looked up at him surprised and he smiled at me. "I've seen you eat ice cream, so I've assumed you had sex."

I laughed, jumped out of my seat and ran around the table to hug him. My mother came down stairs at that exact moment.

My father winked at me and patted my mother on the behind. "Guess what our lovely daughter has been up to?" he asked her in a light, playful voice. My heart nosedived into my stomach. She turned her soft hazel eyes on me and smiled warmly.

"What have you been up to?"

I swallowed hard and looked at my father for courage. He nodded at me while my mother walked over to the counter to fix herself a cup of coffee.

"Mom," I began and then paused. I was starting to shiver as fear wrapped around my chest. "Mom, I'm pregnant."

My mother stopped pouring the coffee and placed the pot and the cup back on the counter. "What did you say?"

"I said, I-- I'm pregnant," I stuttered. I forced myself to lock onto her gaze. There was a storm of emotion swirling under her lashes—shock and disbelief morphed into hurt and disappointment and finally anger.

"You're getting an abortion," she said softly before walking back upstairs. Her bedroom slammed like a clap of thunder. I flinched at the sound and tears sprung to my eyes.

My father patted my hand. "It will be okay," he mumbled. "I'll talk to her." He pushed away from the table, stood, stretched and went upstairs.

***

I sat in the back of a cab between my mother and father staring at my hands. Harry had screamed at me on the phone for two hours straight the night before.

"You're gonna murder my baby because your mother told you to." He repeated that statement twenty or thirty times during our phone conversation. Now it was playing in my head ever and over.

We walked through a crowd of protesters carrying horrifying signs of dead infants. My mother wrapped her arm around my shoulder as we walked through the thickest part of the mob. I will experience this three more times, but I'll only talk about this trip in this book.

After we were signed in and taken to the back. I stripped and put on the hospital gown as instructed. The doctor rapped on the door lightly.

"Are you decent?"

"Yes," I said softly.

She came in the room with my parents close on her heels. I laid back and started to cry. She performed the ultrasound and I started to feel small flutters in my stomach. It was as if the baby was saying, I'm here. I'm here. I let out a low moan that sounded like it came from a wounded animal instead of a young girl.

The doctor stood up and wiped the goop off of my stomach. She looked at my parents and then walked around the table so she could look in my eyes. "If you don't want to do this, you don't have to."

My mother made a gargling sound as if a scream was caught in her throat.

The doctor wiped my tears. "If you say no, then it's no."

"No," I whispered.

"Then, no it is."

It took my mother three months to start speaking to me again.

***

Pregnancy is a wonderful gift and a dreadful curse to someone inflicted with an eating addiction. I had an excuse to overeat and plenty of people willing to feed me. The months rolled on and before I had a chance to realize the gravity of the situation. I was on a delivery table in Hahnemann Hospital undergoing an emergency Caesarian because my pelvic bone ligaments did not soften for childbirth.

On June 23, 1993, after eleven hours of labor, I gave birth to a beautiful baby boy—my greatest achievement to date.

I stayed in the hospital for two weeks after the procedure, suffering every complication known to (wo)man. The nurses would bring my bundle of joy into the room while I slept and I would take him right back to the nursery when I woke up. I was scared to death of the kid, and absolutely terrified to be alone with him.

I had an acute case of postpartum depression. I did not know it at the time. My family dismissed it as the "baby blues," but it was much worse than that. I was afraid of my son. I was afraid of my bedroom. I felt horribly alone and inadequate, and I ate constantly. The depression compounded my eating disorder and I ate morning, noon and night. It stopped adding to my figure, and started accumulating around my midsection. Months had passed and I still looked heavily pregnant.

Harry dropped out of high school and took a job washing dishes to help support our son. Everything that I needed for my son came from someone else. I could do nothing for him. I should have never had him,

I thought one dark day. I hated myself for thinking such a thing. Something was clearly wrong with me, but nobody could see it and I was too ashamed to tell anyone.

The violence in our relationship had grown by leaps and bounds. I started to resent everyone, especially my parents. My father continued his affair, and my mother continued to be oblivious. The depression, resentment, and growing sickness brought on a string of bad decisions that I will outline here.

1)   I transferred out of Strawberry Mansion High to Audenried High School in my twelfth grade year because they had a program for teenage moms and my son could attend school with me. I did this on my own, because I felt I was grown.

2)   I moved in with Harry. My home life had become unbearable—the miserable silence, deceit and loneliness had reached a frightening crescendo.

3)   I dropped out of high school completely a few months after I moved in with Harry. I remember struggling to get my son together for school. He was being difficult and I was depressed over a fight I had the night before with his father. I decided to sit down on the sofa and watch Jerry Springer. When it was

over I noticed that no one was yelling at me to get ready for school. It was in that moment I knew I wasn't going back.

CRITERIASCRITERIASCRITERIASCRITERIASCRITERIASCRITERIASCRITERIAS

-Watch What You Drink

I never realized the amount of calories that I consume on a daily basis when I'm quenching my thirst. This includes my morning coffee routine, the drinks I have for lunch and dinner or when going out for the evening. I take in a lot of empty calories via the drink so I had to take drastic measures to remedy this. Well, there isn't really any drastic measure taking going on, I just liked the way that sound. The following is the drinks I'm going to avoid and why...

Soda

Harvard School of Public Health (HSPH) reports there is a strong link between the consumption of soda and weight gain. Soft drinks are simply liquid candy, and the good people over at onecanofsoda.com have done the math. Those in charge of making the stuff have known this for quite some time, which is why diet sodas were invented. What most people do not realize is that even diet sodas are not good for you. *The carbonation is difficult for your body to process and the sugar substitutes can wreak havoc on your system. I got caught up with the "energy drinks" and "health drinks," too, but I wasn't getting healthy. I was just feeding into a money-making scheme and paying for fancy bottles of syrup. *Health drinks are usually loaded with not only sugar, but preservatives as well. They are money makers for those who want to cash in on the latest health craze.

Coffee

I like a cup of coffee in the morning – who doesn't? But when you load it up with sugar, cream and coffee syrup, you no longer have a cup of coffee, but a calorie-laden dessert. If you want a cup of coffee or a cup of tea in the morning, do yourself a favor and drink it black. If you dislike the taste of the tea or coffee without sugar and cream, then why the heck are you drinking it? *You should limit your coffee and tea consumption to one cup per day as too much caffeine gives you a false high and ends up sending your blood sugar crashing. Also, coffee is very acidic and difficult on the stomach. If you cannot stomach coffee or tea without sugar or cream, you should switch to water!

Juices

Fruit juices are mostly sugar. I used to think that cranberry juice was really good for you, until I read the label. You are actually better off consuming the whole fruit or taking a vitamin supplement. Don't get caught up in drinks that make great health claims, like pomegranate juice, either. While they may contain some healthy compounds, they're mostly made up of sugar and there have been no scientific studies that prove that they have any true health benefits.

Cocktails

Alcoholic drinks are loaded with sugar and can help you pack on the pounds. We often think beer is the alcoholic drink to avoid when dieting. Although beer is loaded with sugars and calories, many wines actually top beer when it comes to sugars.

Drinks I'm going to have

- Water (what a concept)
- Smoothies with frozen, no sugar added fruit. It won't water down your smoothie, there's lots of fiber and it's pretty cost effective.
- Green tea (unsweetened and home brewed, not bottled)
- Coffee (one cup a day without cream or sugar - I don't want to torture you)

Water is like the magic pill for diets. Drinking water is not only good for you, it will boost your metabolism and help you lose weight. We need water to survive. Most people, however, do not drink enough water during the course of the day and get a little dehydrated at times. If you have ever felt thirsty, this is a sign of dehydration. If you drink 6 to 8 glasses of water each day, you will boost your metabolism and aid in weight loss. Once you get used to drinking water, you will also find that it tends to keep you healthier as it flushes toxins out of your system. You can drink green tea, unsweetened, either cold or hot. You should brew it yourself at home because when you purchase bottles of this drink in the store, it is usually loaded with sweeteners and artificial preservatives that totally negate any health advantages of the drink.

Chapter 5 – Temporary Insanity

"Tabitha lost her mind on a sunny Wednesday in May." This is the first line of my debut novel Strawberry Mansion: A Philadelphia Story. I remember writing it. I was sitting in the corner of our small apartment, desperately scribbling on a notepad that was quickly becoming drenched with my tears. Harry had returned home after being gone for an entire week. We argued, he hit me and left again.

This was my life. I traded a bad situation at home for something far worse and writing was the only way to express the constant hell my life had become.

Strawberry Mansion's first chapter displayed Tabitha losing control and stabbing her daughter's father to escape his abuse. My reality was quite different.

I slipped in and out of sanity on a regular basis, and although I'd admit that the abuse was the main cause, his infidelity was also a major factor. Harry began to cheat on me soon after our son was born. I blamed it on my weight gain and bad attitude, but in hindsight I can admit that we were just too young and our relationship was too chaotic.

Over the winter, we had a string of bad storms. I went to visit my older brother in New Jersey and was stranded by an ugly blizzard. There were twenty inches of snow and all public transportation was down. My brother's girlfriend didn't want me and my son to stay with them and she made that shit very evident. A week passed before I could get back to Philly and I vowed that I would never visit my brother again. When I got to my apartment, I was relieved. I tried to kiss Harry, but he pushed me away.

He pointed to the mess in the living room. "This shit better be cleaned up before I get home," he said with a snarl.

Home sweet home...

I just sighed, turned on the music, and started cleaning to the beat. I was too happy to be out of New Jersey to be mad at his bad attitude. I finished up the living room and was about to start on the bathroom when the phone rang. "Hello," I said, turning down the volume on the radio.

"Hey, Moe, you done cleaning up my mess?"

"Who is this?" I asked softly, but I already knew the answer.

"Aw, I'm hurt. I thought you would know my voice by now." She laughed.

"Toya?" I asked as dread flooded my system. "How did you get this number?"

"Don't ask dumb questions, bitch. How do you think I got this number? My man gave it to me when I came over. We fucked and sucked all over that apartment."

"You're a fucking liar," I screamed into the phone before slamming it onto the receiver. Terror tied my stomach into knots. I clutched my chest as tears sprung to my eyes. "You're a fucking liar," I repeated. The phone rang again but I just stared at it. The answering service can pick that shit up, I thought. I don't have time for her lies. Harry cheated on me constantly, but Toya was the only girl I ever really worried about.

Harry spent a lot of time with her, but I had no real proof. The phone started to ring again and fire started to burn away the hurt and replace it with rage. "Look, I know you weren't here, so just stop the bullshit!"

Toya laughed. "You have white furniture in the living room with a flower pattern. The walls are painted gray and the woodwork is white. There are blue fish over top of your clawfoot tub, and matching blue mats and toilet covers. Your son's room is green with a train and car border. Your kitchen is black and white. You want me to tell you what's in your closets?"

I dropped the phone and looked around my tiny apartment, traumatized. A wave of nausea over took and I ran to the bathroom to throw up. The tears came hot, hard and fast. She was here, I thought over and over. He brought her here.

I want to tell you that I packed my bags and left, but I didn't. I want to tell you that I confronted him when he came home, but I didn't. I pulled myself together, washed my face and finished cleaning the house. I made dinner and ate it all by myself. I smoked a pack of cigarettes and made dinner again. I disconnected the phone from the line, because Toya wouldn't stop calling, and I couldn't pretend it was all a lie if I continued to hear her voice.

I pushed the whole conversation to the back of my mind and it was in May that everything exploded. I spent my days tottering between thoughts of homicide and suicide. I was tired of being hit, raped and disrespected. The lines of reality and fantasy blurred more often than not. I had to leave. I needed to get out, but I didn't have anywhere to go. My mother told me that if I walked out of her door, I could not come home. I had no friends, no family and no options. I called Harry's mom, and she told me about a women's shelter downtown.

I spent one horrible night in the shelter and my parents came and got me in the morning. I want to tell you that everything was okay after that, but I can't. I was a mess. I left him for a time. I had a few bad relationships with a few bad men. My self-esteem wasn't low, it was nonexistent. I was naive and looking for love between my legs. Thankfully it didn't take me long to figure out that I was fucking for hugs. I stopped all of the promiscuous behavior after that revelation.

Fucking for hugs, a flaw that I attributed to the character Shanice in Strawberry Mansion, had become my norm. I went back to Harry because I believed he was the only man who would ever love me. I didn't know that you must first love yourself to recognize love from someone else. We were married in the summer of 2000.

Six months later I left him and went to stay with my parents. We were grown and I was tired of him putting his hands on me. I was only trying to make a statement though; I was not prepared to really leave him. I would drive by our house looking for his car, but he was rarely home. On one such drive by, I didn't find his car but decided to go inside anyway to get a fan. My mother kept the heat on hell in the winter and I was finding it hard to sleep.

The door didn't open when I put the key in the lock. I frowned. Someone has to be in here for the bolt to be locked, I thought angrily. My blood started to boil. Banging on the door didn't get me too far, so I stopped. I ran to my car and drove it around the corner. I hopped out with it still running and walked back on my block just in time to see Harry poke his head out of our bedroom window. "You no-good motherfucking bastard."

I went berserk, pounding on the door and screaming at the top of my lungs. I picked up rocks off the street and hurled them at the window. I was getting inside that house by any means necessary.

Harry finally came to the door. "Why don't you stop before someone calls the police?"

"Let me in my house or I guarantee you the police will be here."

"I can't do that," he said softly.

"Hell if you can't. Who do you have in our house, Harry? Who is in the house I grew up in, the house my parents gave us as a wedding gift?"

He shrugged. "A trick."

I screamed and charged at him with everything that was in me. He fell backwards and I raced inside the house. I headed straight for the kitchen and grabbed a steak knife out of the top drawer. I noticed that the back door was open. I cracked my neck and prepared to gut the trick like a fish.

Harry ran into the kitchen and blocked the back door. "What do you think you're gonna do with that?"

I swung the knife wide, slicing his shirt and his arm. He grabbed his arm and moved out of my way. I ran into the backyard and spotted Harry's trick hiding behind the trash can.

"I'm pregnant," she shouted as I started towards her.

All of my anger faded away. I dropped the knife and walked back inside of the house. I had no fight left. I couldn't even understand how my broken heart had the strength to keep beating. I walked around the house in a daze. I couldn't think straight. When the trick came into the living room, I cringed. What kind of women sleeps in another woman's bed? I looked around at the wedding photos hanging on the wall, and shrugged. It didn't matter, nothing mattered. I walked over to the book shelf and picked up little knick-knacks given to me by family members, because I didn't want Harry or his whore to touch them. My arms were full as I blinked away tears and started to head upstairs, when the most devastating thought occurred to me. He expects me to leave. I dropped everything in my hands and turned to face him. I was his wife, yet he was making no attempts to comfort me and kick her out. I walked over to Harry and laughed despite myself. "You want me to leave, don't you?"

He cleared his throat. His eyes darted from me to her and then settled on his hands. "What do you want to do?"

I thought I could not be hurt anymore but I was so wrong. I opened my mouth to respond and bitter salty tears slid inside. "Ask me to leave. You obviously don't want me to be here." I looked around. "Ask me to leave, please," I whispered and was instantly mad at myself. My spine stiffened and I stuck my chin in the air stubbornly. "Everything you've ever done to me, no matter how bad, I always forgave you. I always...I always let you come back. Give me something to hold onto. Ask me to leave my parents' house."

He looked at the girl before meeting my eyes. "I think you should leave, Moe," he said softly.

I nodded and left. I didn't want anything to do with him and that house. I moved in with my parents permanently and promptly ate myself into the hospital.

CRBOCRBOCRBOCRBOCRBOCRBOCRBOCRBO

I have wasted years of my life avoiding daily exercise of any kind. But trying to lose weight, any amount of weight, without exercise is a colossal waste of time. The good news about exercise is that it happens to be the "magic" potion that you need not only to lose weight, but also to maintain good physical and mental health. The bad news is that I have zero staying power.

Each New Year's Eve, I resolve to join a gym with the intent to "get healthy" after bingeing incessantly during the holiday season. I'll even purchase expensive exercise equipment and the latest fitness DVD, but by March, I have given up on the gym and the DVDs. Working out on my home equipment continues to dwindle and eventually drop off completely. The elliptical trainer is little more than a clothes hanger until January when the entire process starts again. *John Tierney published "Be it Resolved" in the New York Times, and reading it let me know I was not alone. The article points out that most people do not keep their resolutions to make healthy life choices because of a state of mental fatigue called "ego depletion." Roy F. Baumeister, a social psychologist at Florida State University, concluded that the way to combat ego depletion and keep your New Year's resolutions was to anticipate the limits of your will power.

Here are some basic strategies to combat ego depletion found on Websites like shanedietresorts.com.

1. SET A SINGLE CLEAR GOAL
2. PRECOMMIT
3. OUTSOURCE
4. KEEP TRACK
5. DON'T OVERREACT TO A LAPSE
6. TOMORROW IS ANOTHER TASTE
7. REWARD OFTEN

The reason that I fail to incorporate exercise into my lifestyle for the long term is simple: I tend to overdo it when I start out. In an effort to lose weight and see results as soon as possible, I forget to warm up and cool down properly and also end up overexerting and injuring myself. This defeats the purpose of exercise, as I am usually laid up in bed while muscles heal. It took me a while to realize that I did not have to buy equipment or join a gym to exercise. I can do this right in the privacy of my own home, or close to home, simply by understanding the importance of activity as well as how cardiovascular exercise and stretching can work.

You have probably heard that you should not exercise close to bedtime or right after a meal. This is true when it comes to cardiovascular exercises, which are designed to get your circulatory system pumping and allow you to burn fat. You do not want to do this before bed as it will give you a burst of energy that may make it difficult for you to fall asleep. There is different heart rate zones used for different kinds of fitness goals.

When I think of cardio a dozen images pop up in my head from Richard Simmons' "Sweating to the Oldies," to Billy Blanks' "TaeBo," and I feel defeated before I begin. Dealing with a food addiction and the waves of shame and depression it brings on can be too much to bear. Taking a brisk walk around the block in the morning before you go to work will get your metabolism working right away and help you burn fat throughout the day. If you are not a morning person, you can do this on your lunch break or when you get home from work. A brisk walk is a great, low-impact way to perform cardiovascular exercise. *Scientists at the University of Pittsburgh recently revealed that overweight people who walked briskly for 30 to 60 minutes a day lost weight even if they didn't change any other lifestyle habits.

Get into a routine when it comes to exercise and make it easy on yourself. Start out slowly and gradually build up your routine. As the pounds start to come off and you feel better about how you look, you will start to look forward to your routine and will also be able to increase your level of activity. Not only will you be able to lose weight, but you will feel more energized throughout the day.

If you are planning on running or doing strenuous exercise, make sure that you warm up first by doing a series of stretching exercises. This will get your muscles ready for exercise and decrease the chances of injury. A few months ago I went walking with a group of women determined to become more active. We were having a good time talking and walking until we came across a group of women jogging and out of the blue I decided to join them—I was so sore the next day, I could barely walk. Please remember to stretch before and after you walk, jog or run. If you don't, you could be in for a world of hurt.

Exercise can also be used as a way to relax you so that you get a good night's sleep. Many people today are so stressed that they complain of trouble sleeping. Take a few minutes each night to do some stretching and some yoga exercises and you will feel more relaxed before bed time and will get a better night's sleep. While we are on the subject of sleeping, it is also a good idea to try to maintain a regular sleeping schedule when you are trying to lose weight. This is actually a good idea for anyone. You should try to go to bed around the same time each night and wake up the same time each morning. This is good for your internal body clock and will aid in regulating your metabolism. *Chris D. Meletis, ND, highlights a study that links sleep loss to weight gain.

Chapter 6 – FUCKING UP ROYALLY

Harry was my husband, the first man I slept with and the father of my child. Getting over him wasn't easy, but I managed. When we broke up the first time, being with another man was the only thing on my young mind. I wanted to get back at him. I wanted to show him that someone else would love to have me. I only hurt myself.

When our marriage ended I was a young adult. I didn't want to jump into another relationship. I wanted to try to find me. I knew I was no longer Moe. Moe was a frightened and lonely little girl. I was becoming Julia, but I didn't know what Julia wanted or what she needed.

On the road to getting right, we often fuck up, and I turned fucking up into an art form. A few years prior to getting married, I went to school to become a medical assistant. I couldn't get a job as a medical assistant to save my life. I did, however, manage to get a job as a care nurse at an institution for mental health, but I was in such emotional turmoil I couldn't hold on to it. I made an error that caused me to get fired. I was in shock when it happened.

I had just made lunch for my residents and sat down to watch "Terminator 2: Judgment Day." They called me upstairs in the office and fired me on the spot. I went downstairs and finished watching the movie. No one rushed me to leave. I think they were afraid I was going to go postal. As soon as the movie was over, I got up from the couch, popped it out of the VCR and left without saying a word to anybody.

I walked all the way home from West Philly. I didn't know how to tell my mother I got fired. I knew my father wouldn't mind, but my mother was a different story. Our relationship was fractured and I didn't want to disappoint her in any way. I got up every day and left the house as if I were going to work. I would go to the bookstore and get lost in fiction. My heart was still aching over Harry. I wrote a host of poetry and short plays as a result of the overload of pain.

A former co-worker called to see how I was doing. She asked if I had filed for unemployment. I told her I didn't know how so she walked me through the steps. She said it was a good time for me to go back to school, but I wasn't ready for that. I was deep into the underground art scene in Philadelphia, performing at any and every open mic that I could find.

I met a young man (let's call him Ricky). He was a music producer who was struggling to get his music off the ground. I was attracted to this dude on a chemical level, but I was still so heartsick and afraid to get hurt. We decided to start a company together. We called it Regal Records (I got a thing for royalty). We worked together constantly. We had great big dreams and enough drive to pull it off, until we slept together.

We couldn't do anything but sleep together after that. Anywhere, at any given moment, we were boning. I started smoking weed and drinking on the regular. My life was spiraling out of control, but I was so caught up in the feeling that I didn't notice it. I was completely self-absorbed, and I liked it. Life was good as far as I was concerned. It was exciting. I was an artist in love with an artist, but he wasn't in love with me. He was in love with his music, and the deeper I fell for him the less concerned I became with that. We were making love every day, five times a day. I was dickmotized.

He noticed it and tried to pull away, right about the same time I got pregnant. This is when reality slapped the fuck out of me. I want to color this part of my life with some sort of magical paint so it won't seem so ugly. I surely didn't want to include this part in the book, but it has to do with my food addiction. At this point you should see the pattern in full bloom. My addiction took a turn for the worse whenever I went through something painful. I was used to getting my ass whooped like Farrah Fawcett in the movie Burning Bed, but I never knew pain like this...

"What do you mean; you want me to get an abortion?" I asked tearfully. I felt so small.

"Julie, neither one of us is working. I just had a son that I can barely take care of. Having another kid just doesn't make sense right now—for either of us."

I couldn't breathe. I started to panic. My heart was racing and tiny beads of sweat broke out on my forehead. I held the phone receiver with both hands. I didn't want to hear another word from him, but I didn't have the strength to hang up the phone.

"Look, ma, we're not even together. Having an abortion is the only real option."

I dropped the phone and ran outside. I needed air. I needed to think. I was at the end of my unemployment benefits and living at home with my parents and young son. How did I get here? What was I going to do? I threw up all over my mother's garden.

I wiped my mouth on my sleeve and broke out into a run. I ran as fast as I could, breathing hard and pushing hard. I collapsed in a park twenty blocks from my house. I sat under a tree and hugged my knees close to my chest. He doesn't want me, and he damn sure doesn't want this baby, I thought over and over. It took me five hours to cry myself dry, and three more hours to find the strength to get up. I went home and drank a half a bottle of vodka. I was going to have an abortion, because the thought of having a second child on my own without a job was beyond frightening.

Once I made an appointment to have the procedure done, I felt hollow. I would look at women with their small children and cringe. I was a coward. I walked around like a zombie eating everything in sight. My second go-round at the abortion clinic was much like the first.

The horrible mob of the protesters out front of the clinic was hard to get through by myself, but I managed. I sat in that office looking in the faces of the other women in the room. What's your story? I wondered. When Ricky walked in the door I felt a little relief, but not that much. Everything about the visit to the abortion clinic is etched into my soul. I can tell you what the doctor looked like; I can describe the paintings on the wall and the aseptic smell of the room. All the feelings I had for Ricky died that day.

We broke up shortly after that. I crawled into my son's bed every night to hold him and watch him sleep. I would cry a lot. He came in my room one day and smiled at me. "You should stop being sad, Mommy. You've been sad long enough."

Out of the mouths of babes…

I wanted to be strong for my son. I wanted him to respect me, so I learned how to respect myself. I stopped dressing provocatively because I didn't like the attention anymore. I went back to school and started looking for a job. I wanted to be someone my son could look up to. I wanted desperately to regain my self-worth. A couple of years floated by and I was starting to heal. I even stopped overeating and lost some weight.

I focused on my son and everything else in my life was starting to line up. I couldn't find work in the medical field so I took a job at a call center for PECO energy. Not the best job in the world, but it beat the hell out of a zero. You know what they say about finding love when you stop looking…

That's exactly how it happened, but I wasn't ready. I wish I knew that. I wish someone would have told me.

CRUORCRUORCRUORCRUORCRUORCRUORCRUORCRUO

-Putting it All Together

So, now you are ready to start your own weight loss journey. You already know what foods and drinks you have to avoid and you should have some sort of exercise routine planned to increase your level of activity. Here are some tips on what you can eat throughout the day to keep yourself nourished:

Breakfast

This is actually where you want to consume the most calories. There is an old saying; "Eat breakfast like a king, eat lunch like a prince, and eat dinner like a pauper." *Tricia Cunningham, who co-wrote "The

Reverse Diet" with Heidi Skolnik, MS, CDN, FACSM, recommends switching breakfast and dinner as part of a weight loss program. According to Cunningham, approximately 100,000 people across the country are eating their dinner for breakfast and losing weight. Although I am not a fan of switching the food, I am in total agreement with switching my caloric intake and consuming most of my calories in the morning. Breakfast ideas for a diet include cereal that is unsweetened such as Special K and Cheerios. Measure the cereal into a bowl and watch your calorie intake. Use skim milk for your cereal and, if possible, add fresh fruit. Blueberries are not only low in calories when compared to other fruits, but they are also very nutritious and high in antioxidants.

Eggs are often criticized for being high in cholesterol, but they are an excellent source of protein. You can have an egg for breakfast as long as you cook it properly. Soft boiled eggs are good as are hard boiled eggs.

If you like toast, you can eat a slice of whole grain wheat toast with fruit preserves or a little butter (natural fat in small amounts is not bad). Use a teaspoon to measure the preserves so that you do not indulge too much.

Oatmeal is very good if you choose rolled or steel cut oats over instant oatmeal. It's high in fiber and can be sweetened with fresh berries, and apple slices. Oatmeal is very good for maintaining good cholesterol; it is filling and works well to get your morning started off on the right foot.

Skip the breakfast bars. They are high in sugar, preservatives and fat. If you truly do not want to take time to make breakfast and eat it at home, then take a banana with you on your way to work. A nutrition bar has about 250 calories; a banana has about 70 calories.

Snack

Have a mid-morning snack. You can have a number of different things, but they should be measured and the calories counted. An apple is a good source of vitamins, takes a few minutes to eat and can be filling. Be sure to drink plenty of water throughout the morning to continue to keep your metabolism going. Many so called healthy snack packs like trail mixes are actually very high in calories. Unsalted sunflower seeds are a good source of protein. A mid-morning snack will take the edge off of your hunger and help you so that you do not overindulge in your lunch.

Lunch

Leafy green salads with a lean protein like grilled chicken, steak or tuna are good for lunch. Your lunch should be something that you brought from home or a salad at a local restaurant. Try using vinegar and oil to dress your salad instead of ranch, as it is lower in calories. If you can, try eating a salad with just vinegar or splashes of lemon. I did this once for a week and lost five pounds without doing anything else. Vinegar has hardly any calories at all.

Oranges are a good source of nutrition and can be good for after lunch. The sweet flavor of the orange will top off the meal and give you a feeling of satisfaction and because they take a while to peel, this will also keep you from being tempted into eating more. Again, you will want to continue drinking water throughout the day, especially with your meals.

Low fat cottage cheese or, better yet, ricotta cheese, is an excellent source of protein and can be eaten for lunch. The same is true with low-fat yogurt, but please remember to check your labels, because some products add a ridiculous amount of sugar in place of fat. You have a variety of choices when it comes to your lunch and you can have up to 400 calories. At the end of lunch, you should not still feel hungry.

Snack

Although people scoff at "rabbit food" diets, raw celery and carrots are not only good for you, but they have hardly any calories at all. When you are snacking after lunch, be sure to stay away from salty snacks such as crackers, as they can cause you to retain water. You will notice the weight starting to come off in the first two days of the diet, although much of this will be water weight. You will also notice that you will be making more trips to the bathroom. This is good as you are flushing toxins from your system.

Dinner

You want to keep your calories down during dinner and it should be your last meal of the day. You will find that the more you eat in the morning, the less you will need to eat for dinner. You can have a normal dinner with the family, just watch the portions. Keep your calorie intake to the limit and skip dessert. Be mindful of how the meal is cooked. Substitute olive oil for other fats and broil, poach or steam your foods instead of other frying or sautéing.

One way that you can enjoy dinner without feeling as though you are depriving the entire family as well as yourself is to simply cut your portions in half.

Drink a glass of water before the meal, eat slowly and chew your food more instead of wolfing it down. This will take you longer to eat and will allow you to feel content in a shorter period of time.

You should, after each meal or snack, feel satisfied and not stuffed. Many people feel that in order to be satisfied with a meal, they have to feel full. You do not want to feel as you are bursting at the seams, you simply do not want to feel hungry. By understanding how many calories you are consuming as compared to how many you need, you have a leg up on losing weight. The more you are aware of the calories in the foods that you are eating and the foods that you need to avoid, the easier dieting will become.

Chapter 7 – MARRIED: THE SEQUEL

To paint my second husband in a purely negative light would be the worst kind of deception. He's not an evil man. He is a good person with a good heart, and our marriage was filled with happiness in the beginning. However, our demons won out in the end.

We met in the spring of 2004. I started to perform poetry again and he was in the reserves. My soldier. He was well-versed in history and theology. We would talk on the phone for hours about politics and religion. He took me to nice restaurants and for long walks through the park. He always treated me like a lady and called me his Queen. I had never been courted before. It was nice. He invited me up to Harrisburg to meet his family. I was nervous as hell and felt so out of place. His parents were different from the people I was used to, and I didn't know how to take them. Although, his father obviously knew how to take me: he called me ghetto the very first time I met him and implied that I was after his son's money.

I was tempted to slap the shit out of him, but knew that would only solidify the whole ghetto image. His mom and his sister did their best to smooth things over and make me feel welcome, but the damage was done and the line was drawn. His father put me on the defensive with his statements and I stayed there. The urge to bitch slap his father remained strong; however, I didn't want to go to jail, so I didn't say anything. I walked down to the rec room and told his son I was ready to go.

It took six months for me to introduce him to my son. We moved in together a year after that. I was very happy and very blind. I fell for this man with no safety net, because I had become addicted to his gentle touch and focused attention. I followed him to his hometown of Harrisburg and left everything I knew behind. Before I realized the gravity of my decision, I was already drowning in my emotions. He was activated in the military and stationed in Fort Dix. The loneliness that plagued my childhood bubbled to the surface, and I ate everything I could get my hands on. I gained 40 pounds in four months--gorging on food after my son went to bed at night and before he woke up in the morning.

Harrisburg was turning into my personal hell, but had the opposite effect on my son. He prospered in the excellent Susquehanna Township school system. He made friends and socialized for the first time in his young life. I desperately wanted to go home, but I couldn't rob him of this experience. My son was getting the childhood I never had, so I stayed when everything inside me told me to go.

I moved to Harrisburg in the summer of 2005 and came home broken in the summer of 2009. My years there had completely changed my outlook on life. In keeping with the theme of this book, I won't chronicle my entire HBG experience, but I will highlight the breaking point as it relates to my addiction.

After being medically discharged from the service, my second husband (let's call him Bruce) found it hard to find a job, and harder still to keep one. The transition from military life from a civilian existence is a bitch and a half. My wages were not enough to sustain our lifestyle and we started to fall miserably behind. Both sets of our parents offered assistance to shore up our mounting debt, but it was little more than one single dose of Pepto against a major case of the shits and we were sinking fast. Bruce would not agree to downgrade. We were living well above our means and I started to work day and night to compensate. My logic was pure and simple. This man took care of me when he could. He bought me a car and provided a beautiful apartment, so I was not about to leave his side in his time of need. I was determined to do whatever it took to make a way for us.

One of the nurses at my job told me I was going to kill myself with the hours I was working. She convinced me to enroll in nursing school. "No matter how you sling it, Julia, nine dollars an hour is nine dollars an hour. Invest in your future or you are going to look up twenty years from now and find yourself in the same spot." I took her words to heart and hit the books like they were going to fight back. After a long discussion with Bruce, he decided to go back to school as well. The GI Bill would provide and, if we were careful, we could make it.

We were not careful.

I excelled in school. I had a 4.0 GPA and was accepted into the college's highly competitive nursing clinical program. Clinicals were demanding and I found it hard to keep up with my studies and work full time. The financial strain started to show in our relationship. I didn't want to quit because I was so close to finishing. In two semesters, I would be a nurse and financially secure. I asked Bruce to drop out of school since he had much longer to reach his degree.

"In a few short months, I will be able to take care of everything, and then you can go to school full time."

He looked at me and sneered. "That's stupid. What would I look like working two jobs?"

That question pierced my heart. I felt as if he just punched me in the face. You would look like me, I thought. I worked eighty hours a week until I started school, and worked sixty hours with a full class load. I walked into the bathroom so he wouldn't see my tears.

The last couple of weeks of class were the worst. I couldn't focus to save my life. I would get out of lecture and go straight to work. After work, I would sit up at my computer for hours crying and trying to make sense of my assignment. One night my son got up to go to the bathroom and heard my tears. He came over to my desk and hugged me. He wiped my tears away and smiled.

"Why are you going to school to be a nurse, Mom? All you do is write."

Now that question fucked my world straight up. When I finally left school it was a relief. I was going to finish Strawberry Mansion and become a world famous author (still trying to work that out).

The rift between me and Bruce grew every day. I dropped out of college and he stayed in. I took on a second job and he quit his. We received an eviction notice in December of that year, and I decided that I had had enough. I was tired of making a way. I was tired of his cavalier attitude. He didn't care to be a provider anymore and was constantly looking to me to lead us out of trouble.

I went home to visit my parents for the holidays and decided I wasn't going back. I was tired, depressed and miserable. I gained a whopping 85 pounds to prove it. Bruce came to Philadelphia and apologized. He told me that he took care of everything and he needed his wife by his side. He made sweet, gentle love to me and assured me that everything was going to be different. He said that he got a loan from his father and a new job.

He lied.

I went back to Harrisburg happier then I had been in a long time. I got hired at a nursing home called Spring Creek, and I liked it. For a very brief time, things were really looking up.

Then we were evicted. We had to move in with his mother until we could find a place to stay. I worked every day sixteen hours a day, so that I could buy a house. I caught a cold, and still worked. It morphed into bronchitis and I still worked. Then it turned into pneumonia, but I still worked. I worked until I passed out and had to be hospitalized. I purchased a house on Holly Street and we moved in shortly after being discharged from the hospital.

In the back of my mind, I knew that Bruce no longer loved me. Our relationship changed after the first day I left him and it never healed. A few months after we moved in to our new home, I found out that Bruce was still receiving a substantial amount of money from the military each month. He let me work myself to death's doorstep without blinking an eye. I got up from the computer and looked at my reflection. My hair was pulled up into a matted ponytail. I was 336 pounds and suffering from diabetic neuropathy from drinking and overeating — most days I could barely walk.

"You're gonna die here, Moe," I whispered softly to my reflection. "If you stay here, you are gonna die." I called my mother, and she brought me home.

CRITECRITECRITECRITECRITECRITECRITECRITE

-To Sum it Up

I did not want to write a book that gives you details on exactly how much to eat and what on which day, as this rarely works. Not everyone has the same tastes when it comes to food and not everyone needs the same amount of calories. The trick is to eat foods that are good for you and will provide you with the nutrition that you need to maintain your body. If the foods that I have listed do not appeal to you, then eat the foods that you normally eat and simply cut the portions in half. Eat breakfast; drink plenty of water and make time to exercise. You will lose the weight if you follow this outline.

• Find out how many calories you need to sustain yourself based on your body type, height, activity level and gender

• Use the sedentary scale for calories you need and cut it by 200

• Eat breakfast!

• Increase your exercise level by performing cardiovascular exercises such as speed walking for at least 10 minutes each day

• Eliminate fast foods, fried foods, processed foods, sweets, and frozen meals from your diet

• Drink water or unsweetened green tea instead of any other drink and avoid alcohol

• Drink 6-8 glasses of water or green tea each day

• Consume steady calories throughout the day instead of all in one meal

When dieting on a long-term basis, it is safe to lose two pounds a week. It is a good idea to keep yourself motivated by giving yourself some sort of reward when you have accomplished your goal.

Remember that if you get sidetracked and end up falling off the wagon, just pick yourself up and get right back on track. Do not beat yourself up over a mishap - it is in the past and there is nothing that you can do to move time backwards. Concentrate on the future and moving forward.

Chapter 8 – HOME AGAIN

For some fucked up reason, I didn't view going home as ending my marriage. I just wanted to get better. I was too sick to go back to work, and I had little faith in Bruce's ability to keep his job. Moving back in with his mother was not an option, at least not for me. Don't get me wrong, his family is lovely, but we had this oil and water thing going on that always made me feel like an uncomfortable outsider.

I truly thought we were going to make it through the situation. I just knew that I was going to get better and we were going to take financial classes, receive marriage counseling, and come out on top.

I held onto that fantasy every time Bruce came to Philly to see me. "He was visiting me because he loved me and he believed me when I said we were going to make it," I said to anyone who asked. I mean really, who drives one hundred miles just to fuck?

I managed to convince myself that our marriage was not over; I was just sick and Bruce actually did love me. My mom nursed me back to health and my agency transferred me to the Philadelphia VA hospital. For the first time I my life I was surrounded by strong, educated and opinionated black women. I never had so many positive role models.

Things were starting to look up.

I was going to work hard, save my money, and Bruce and I and our sons were going to have a brand new start.

Then he stopped returning my calls.

Then I started to see pictures of him and another woman all over the internet.

Then he changed his Facebook status from married to "It's complicated."

Then my cell phone was disconnected.

Then my van was repossessed.

Then, finally, I received the divorce papers in the mail, and even my overactive imagination couldn't stand up to the evidence. He didn't love me anymore and I now had the proof in black and white.

I went to the local wine and spirits and blew my entire paycheck on cheap booze. I spent the next couple of weeks in a self-imposed stupor. I felt way too much, and I didn't want to feel anything. I shut the world out, but a few determined people who loved me climbed over the walls that I erected.

I walked around with the divorce papers in my pocketbook for months. No matter how hard I tried, I couldn't bring myself to sign them. To my horror, I discovered that I was still madly in love with Bruce and I had no idea how not to be. How do you stop loving someone?

This was a very painful time in my life. I was so far from the Julia I am now and nowhere near the Julia that I hope to become. My friend Rachel called me on the phone and had me sign the papers. It took two weeks to mail them off after that. During those days, I never really felt as if my feet were on solid ground. Sometimes I would be perfectly fine and others I was a total fucking mess. In the midst of my storm, at a moment of brief calm, my father left my mother. I came home to see her curled up on her bed crying. She looked so small. I climbed in bed with her. I knew the pain she was going through. I knew it well.

We clung to each other in this dark time. Bit by bit, day by day, we grew a little stronger and the pain began to fade. My son kept me on a strict writing schedule and his father-- yes my first husband-- became my biggest supporter. Harry showed up when I was at my worst. I took a few days off work to suck on a bottle of Mad Dog 20/20 like it was mother's milk. I frowned when I heard a knock on my bedroom door-- no one in my family knocks on my door, they just barge the hell in.

"It's open," I said with a frown. When Harry walked in the room I shot off the bed like a rocket.

"What are you doing here?"

He smiled and those damn dimples popped up. "I just came to see if my son was telling me the truth. I wanted to know if the great Julia Press Simmons had become a lazy lush."

"My son called me a lazy lush?"

He shrugged. "He didn't use those exact words."

"Get the fuck out of my house."

He ignored me and started picking up my booze.

"Get off of my shit. Put that back." I tried to grab the bottles from him but he just snatched them away and called my son, who came in the room with a trash can. My son couldn't meet my eyes as they started throwing my liquor away.

I started to cry. Harry walked over to me and wiped my eyes. "Mook told me how much money you needed to get your books printed. I gave him the money and told him to order the books. What else do you need?"

My heart dropped to my stomach. "I don't want your help," I whispered. "I'm not doing that anymore."

"You're not doing what anymore?"

"Writing. I'm not writing or publishing anymore. I'm tired."

He let out a bitter laugh. "I did horrible things to you. Things I'm ashamed of, things I'll never forgive myself for. It didn't break you, though." He walked to the door. "Who would have thought a piece of paper from a nigga in Harrisburg could snap you in two."

He left me with that thought, and that thought changed everything. I'm not perfect. I'll never be perfect, but I want to be whole. I want to be strong. I want to be free. I made a decision that day. I decided that I'm no longer giving myself permission to hurt myself. I'm not going to run from my problems. I started a journey. It's not easy. I mess up more often than not. I now weigh 280 pounds. I've lost 56 pounds since the day my first husband visited me two years ago. I struggle every day, but I've resolved to be honest about it.

I wrote this book for the people who suffer as I suffer. I hope that by sharing the story of my addiction you will find strength to face yours. I do not assume that everyone is obese for the same reasons. If you are happy with your weight and you are physically healthy, then I am happy for you. However, if you are hurting and you want to change, I hope that this book lets you know that you are not alone. I hope that you find the courage to face your underlying problems head on. I hope that this little book screams to you that

YOU HAVE NO REASON TO BE
ASHAMED!

I couldn't wait to lose the weight to tell my story, because I found the journey, the struggle just as interesting

#FuckitImFat #NotforLong

****

-Falling Down

So what happens when, after a few days, you get tempted with a piece of cake or some other treat? What happens if you wake up late one morning and do not have time to take your walk? In other words, what do you do when you fall off the wagon? You get up, you dust your ass off, and you climb right back on. Many people get discouraged when they fall off the wagon, to the point that they decide that the entire idea has to be scrapped. Fear of failing again can keep them from even trying to continue with the diet or the healthy lifestyle choice that they have made for themselves. So they go back into their familiar routine, despite the fact that it was not working for them.

The world will not stop spinning if you make a mistake while trying to change your lifestyle. You fucked up and ate a piece of cake or didn't exercise for a day - so what? Everyone makes mistakes. This does not mean that you are a failure. Just get right back into the groove and continue with the plan as if nothing happened. Beating yourself up will not help you. One piece of cake will not sabotage your diet. But giving up because you had that piece of cake will destroy all that you worked for.

Do not be afraid of failure. Continue to persist with your healthy lifestyle choice, despite setbacks. Do not view a deviation as a colossal failure, but as a slight setback in what you want to do and continue on with your goal.

THE END & THE BEGINING

In 2005, I was diagnosed with type 2 diabetes. To find out more about this disease here, read the Center for Disease Control's report on Diabetes Mellitus. I want to hear your story, so please write to me at jpresssimmons@gmail.com. I am not a doctor or a dietician, so please seek professional help for all your dieting needs! Want to see how I'm doing? Follow my blog and my journey: www.jpsimmons.com.

SOURCES

METABOLISM

Recommended Reading - Secrets to a Healthy Metabolism by Maria Emmerich

http://www.merriam-webster.com/dictionakry/metabolism

*Harvey, Michele **"Does Your Metabolism Slow Down As You Age"**
http://www.livestrong.com/article/392178-does-your-metabolism-slow-down-as-you-age/#ixzz20Yf3yMxy

*Zeratsky, Katherine R.D., L.D. **"Weight loss"**
https://www.mayoclinic.com/health/metabolism/AN01772

Mayo Clinic Staff **"Metabolism and weight loss: How you burn calories"**
https://www.mayoclinic.com/health/metabolism/WT00006

CALORIE CONSUMPTION

Recommended Reading - The CalorieKing Calorie, Fat & Carbohydrate Counter 2012 by Allan Borushek

http://www.freedieting.com/tools/calorie_calculator.htm

Layton, Julia "How Calories Work"
http://health.howstuffworks.com/wellness/diet-fitness/weight-loss/calorie1.htm

FOODS TO AVOID

Recommended reading: The Lean Belly Prescription by Travis Stork MD and Peter Moore & Lick The Sugar Habit by Nancy Appleton

nutrition.mcdonalds.com/getnutrition/nutritionfacts.pdf

*Hazell, Kyrsty **"Frying Food 'Doesn't Increase Heart Disease Risks' Claims Study"**
http://www.huffingtonpost.co.uk/2012/01/24/frying-food-doesnt-increase-heart-disease-risks_n_1228437.html

*: *BMJ 2012;344:e363*
http://www.bmj.com/content/344/bmj.e363

BMJ. 2012; 344: e363.

http://www.ncbi.nlm.nih.gov/pmc/articles/PMC3265571/

*trans-fat research
http://www.thelabrat.com/review/WhatIsTransFat.shtml

*processed food research
http://www.heart.org/HEARTORG/Conditions/HighBloodPressu re/PreventionTreatmentofHighBloodPressure/Processed-Foods-Where-is-all-that-salt-coming-from_UCM_426950_Article.jsp

Jegtvig, Shereen **"What Are Processed Foods?"**
http://nutrition.about.com/od/askyournutritionist/f/processedfood s.htm

Stacey, **"Is Frozen Food Healthy?"**
http://www.buildingnutrition.com/content/is-frozen-food-healthy/

Dr. Gupta, Sanjay **"Is sugar toxic?"**
http://www.cbsnews.com/8301-18560_162-57407294/is-sugar-toxic/

Sugar's effect on your health
http://www.healingdaily.com/detoxification-diet/sugar.htm

http://www.heart.org/HEARTORG/Conditions/HighBloodPressu re/PreventionTreatmentofHighBloodPressure/Processed-Foods-Where-is-all-that-salt-coming-from_UCM_426950_Article.jsp

DRINKS TO AVOID

Sugary Drinks or Diet Drinks: What's the Best Choice?
http://www.hsph.harvard.edu/nutritionsource/healthy-drinks/sugary-vs-diet-drinks/

How much sugar is in one can of soda?
http://www.onecanofsoda.com/

Bond, Owen **"Health Risks of Carbonated Water"**
www.livestrong.com/article/313171-health-risks-of-carbonated-water/

WHAT I'M EATING

Recommended Reading: Eat, Drink, and Be Healthy [Kindle Edition] **Walter Willett M.D.**

Salomon, Sharon B. MS, RD *"Does eating the largest meal of the day in the morning promote weight loss?"*
http://www.todaysdietitian.com/newarchives/tdjuly2007pg48.shtml

Jennings, Kerri-Ann M.S., R.D. *"Learn how to clean up your diet with these 10 healthy tips."*
http://www.eatingwell.com/

Healthy Eating for Weight Loss Reviewed by Jonathan L Gelfand, MD http://women.webmd.com/guide/nutrition-101-how-to-eat-healthy

EXERCISE

TIERNEY, JOHN **"Be It Resolved"**
http://www.nytimes.com/2012/01/08/sunday-review/new-years-resolutions-stick-when-willpower-is-reinforced.html?pagewanted=all

Sirico, Stephanie **"Use Your Willpower For Weight Loss"**
http://shanedietresorts.com/blog/426/use-your-willpower-for-weight-loss/

Zerbe, Leah **"8 Astonishing Benefits of Walking"**
http://www.rodale.com/benefits-walking

Bee, Peta **"Forget the gym: Why a brisk walk is a really great workout"**
http://www.active.com/walking/Articles/Forget_the_gym__Why_a_brisk_walk_is_a_really_great_workout.htm

SLEEP DEPRIVATION

Meletis, Chris D. ND **"Does sleep loss cause weight gain?"**
http://www.fr.sott.net/articles/show/222880-Does-sleep-loss-cause-weight-gain-

Shomon, Mary **"Sleep More, Lose Weight"**

http://thyroid.about.com/od/loseweightsuccessfully/a/sleepdiet.htm

http://www.webmd.com/sleep-disorders/excessive-sleepiness-10/lack-of-sleep-weight-gain

Understanding Food Addiction

http://www.oa.org/

http://www.fitwoman.com/our-program/special-tracks/understanding-food-addiction/

Ashley N. Gearhardt, MS, William R. Corbin, PhD, and Kelly D. Brownell, PhD **"Food Addiction An Examination of the Diagnostic Criteria for Dependence"**
https://sites.google.com/site/foodaddictionlibrary/collections/research-articles

Queen Midas Books

Presents Other Works By

JULIA PRESS SIMMONS

Strawberry Mansion Series

STRAWBERRY MANSION: A PHILADELPHIA STORY

Nook Strawberry Mansion: A Philadelphia Story

BEGONIA BROWN: A PHILADELPHIA STORY

Nook Begonia Brown: A Philadelphia Story

VIOLET: STRAWBERRY MANSION 3

Nook Violet: Strawberry Mansion 3

Strawberry Mansion The Trilogy

Nook Strawberry Mansion Trilogy

SM4: A Hustler's Heart

Fornication Series

Fornication Volume One

Nook Fornication Volume One

Fornication Volume Two

DAWN OF DESTRUCTION EMini Seriries

This is a serial novel published in chapters

FOLLOW ME ON TWITTER

www.twitter.com/jpsimmons

LIKE ME ON FACEBOOK